Introduction

From the start of the time the main need for mankind was the food, shelter and health. The time passes by and the mankind started to flourish in the world. People started to choose different professions for the survival and to meet the needs for their life. They learned the trade system and in this way the world came into a system. During all of these eras main essential need for the humans was the health. As the human body is made with such complexities that even the human throughout the history cannot find proper medication for the all diseases. We have been continuously striving for the cycle of life.

We do a lot of efforts to make

our lives more beautiful and peaceful. We work day and night to do something for the survival. In the race of life we have come so far that we couldn't understand that where the actual meaning of life is. The most important aspect of life for a human being is health. Everyone in the world is very conscious about their health. As it's a saying health is the wealth. So most precious thing is health, if you are healthy then you have everything, without health there is nothing.

While during this time we are that much advance in all the aspects of life, even in health, but still there is an alarming condition that is also this era's advancement. As human being started to revolutionize it also bring so many catastrophes with him. We are so much busy in our life that we don't have time to take care of ourselves. That is why we do not take any conscious steps regarding our health therefore our health is becoming week day by day.

Chronic pain is the most alarming situation in this era; it has been affecting the people and causing them a very serious situation for the people of all ages. Chronic pain is a pain which remains more than 12 weeks despite doing medication or even the treatment. It is the most common medical issue for people without considering the cause of people or ethnicity or age. It affects the people of middle age especially.

More than 80 percent of the

population of the world is now facing the same issue. We can see that in our surroundings, like office, home, playground, or in any public place. We can find people having same issue of the chronic pain. This pain is not affiliated to a particular part of the body. It is a continuous pain in the body which remains in the body more than some of the weeks.

According to a survey in America more than 110 million of the people are living in America, suffering the same condition of this severe chronic pain. It could be any type of pain like headache, postsurgical pain, post-trauma pain, lower back pain, cancer pain, arthritis pain, neurogenic pain (pain caused by nerve damage), psychogenic pain (pain that isn't caused by disease, injury, or nerve damage).

But from these the most common chronic pain which people are facing are chronic back pain, chronic neck back pain and migraine headaches. So to get the relief from these pains people usually get medications, prescribed and over-the-counter drug. These medications gave the timely relief to the people but this is not the proper treatment. People from the age between 25 to 60 faces these chronic pains more than the younger ones, but it could be at any age even to the younger ones. This chronic pain is like an pandemic which is spreading and there are no measurements taken by the government of any country in the world. As it is a very huge level medical problem rather than other problems.

As it attracts no attentions for the higher authorities therefore there is almost no research going on regarding this chronic pain in the world that is why it does not have any proper treatment. Chronic pain is also very difficult to be located by the medical professional, as for this there is no proper testing, as there is no research on it.

Also in medical schools they even do not pay any attention on the students to teach them that how they can handle this type of pain, how they can locate the pain and what are the measurements which should be taken to treat such patients. The number of the people going through this severe condition is increasing day by day as the population of the world is rapidly increasing day after the day.

As doctors are not properly teach to handle this condition that is a very scary fact. After all going through these tough times still we are trying our best to help the people who are going through this worst condition of pain.

It is advice that not to go to any medical expert or let say any doctor, if you are facing this type of pain. There are many reasons to do so as we will discuss in this book. Here we will discuss that how to locate or let say how can you examine your own self, How can you treat yourself. As due to lack of knowledge about these type of pain people usually ignores these chronic pains which will be of more loss and will do more damage in future.

To handle these types of condition firs of the entire most important thing is to know about these chronic pains. So that you would not fall into the hands of selfish doctors or any other professionals, as they do not have proper knowledge about chronic pain so they will either prescribe you wrong medicines or will give you wrong tests suggestions or they will ask you to visit them for many times so that treatment could be fulfilled.

But in reality they are not helping you, they are helping themselves by selling different medicines or doing unnecessary tests which will cost you much more and the wrong treatment will also affect you in more complicated way.

 That is why you need to improve your knowledge about this chronic pain so that you would not fall into the hands of these fake experts who even do not have proper education in the subject of chronic pain.

That is why in this book we are teaching you proper knowledge and guidelines to do necessary steps to examine the disease and to do proper treatment.

In first chapter we will study about the chronic pain. What are the causes of chronic pain? What are the types of chronic pain in details? How to examine and locate these pains? What is yoga? How to treat these pains with the help of yoga?

After reading this book you will be in the position to do what is best for you. You will also be able the help other people who are suffering from these pains. I am pretty sure you have seen such people who are suffering from these kinds of diseases and they are already having wrong treatment. To do medication is not the sole solution to handle chronic pain. The most effective way to treat these pains is the yoga. As self help is the most effective help in examining and treating yourself.

What is yoga?

 The mental, physical and spiritual practices conducted in such a way that it helps human being to bring peace of mind, satisfaction of spirit and the fitness of body, is called YOGA.

Yoga as an exercise is a physical activity that consists mainly of posture, which is usually linked to a flow sequence, sometimes accompanied by doing breathing exercises, and often ends with resting on the floor or meditation. Yoga in this form is now known all over the world, especially in America and Europe. It is based on the posture used in the ancient spiritual guidance of Haṭha yoga, but is often referred to as "yoga". Scholars have offered yoga as a form of various vocabulary exercises, including contemporary modern yoga and world Anglophone yoga.

It is the interaction between
the body, the spirit and the
god. It helps us to increase
our inner peace and to gain
the wisdom. By the help of
yoga we came to know
more about the life, the
knowledge about the life
and the meaning of the life.
It helps us to connect with
the spirit and with the god. It
helps us to live a both
physical and spiritual
contentment life.

Union between the body,
the mind and God which
helps man attain knowledge
and wisdom and develops
his thought by developing
his knowledge of life; it
protects him from
sectarianism, religious
fanaticism, narrow-
mindedness and
shortsightedness when
searching; it makes him live

a life of contentment both physically and spiritually."

History

 As YOGA has a very rich history of more than 5000 years. So it is not specified that when did the YOGA started and how it came to being in existence. Some scholars believe that the YOGA started from the age of Indus Valley Civilization. It was a civilization which was establish in South Asia, now in the Pakistan their traces are found at the place of Punjab province. Some believe that the origin of yoga started from over there. As we know that those civilizations are being vanished from the places of history and there is no proper knowledge about that civilization that is why we cannot say this exactly that it is true.

 Some references to yoga are between 500BC and 200 BC, it was taken places when philological ideas of Hinduism and Buddhism. As there is a huge difference between experts about the origin of yoga so it is not specified that when does it started and who does started it.

 Here we will get to know about the start of the yoga in different steps from the point where we have proper knowledge, regardless of assumption that how and when does it started.

 Basically it has four different steps of development.

- **Pre- Classic Yoga**
- **Classic Yoga**

- **Post classic Yoga**

- **Modern Yoga**

Pre-Classical Yoga

This was the age of the most ancient civilization every found, named as Indus valley civilization over five thousand years ago. Archaeologists discovered a lot of the pictures like seals containing images of a person sitting in the meditative position. This is the yoga position, from that discovery it is considered to be the first civilization ever to practice yoga for the peace of spirit and the body also the mind.

Its origin is concerned with the

Hinduism and Buddhism. The first citation of the yoga was found in the oldest text of Hinduism named as the Rig Veda. Also keeping in mind all the other things, that Vedas were being transmitted for more than ten thousand years orally or much more than that. Basically the Vedas are the collections of different songs, mantras and rituals in the form of text which were used by so called the Brahmans. These Vedas also contain a very large size of the collection of the science, Nature's mother, mathematics, the agriculture, the social science, morality, ethics, culture, agriculture, the arts and a lot more. Brahmans are considered to be the most sacred and high level cast in Hinduism. These Brahmans were the Vedic priests. The yoga was developed by the Rishis and the Brahmans, in different time periods. It keeps on changing with time by time. Rishis and Brahmans both stored their beliefs and practices in a book, called as Upanishads. The Upanishads is the part of Vedas and the first explicit reference of the yoga was found in it. This contains more than 200 scriptures. In Hinduism the most sacred book Bhagavad Gita, contains most of the Yogic scripts in it.

 It was composed around 500 BCE according to the Hinduism religion. It was written by the great Sage Patanjali around 500 BCE. He wrote the whole process that systematic process of practical methods which are helpful for awaking the higher levels of the mind and also to expand those higher levels of mind. It helps to awake the intellect and the consciousness of the mind. Yoga sutras consist on the 196 lines which were written in Sanskrit and then it is divided into 4 parts. The Upanishads got the idea of sacrifice from the Vedas, that ritual sacrifice teaches the sacrifice of ego through the knowledge and information of the meaning of life. In yoga the most important thing which is being mentioned ever is that the patience, patience in every condition and that patience brings the peace, inner peace. It also teaches the practical yoga and the yoga for the mind. Through the yoga of mind our level of wisdom increases day by day and we came to know about the peace, the inner peace.

Classic Yoga:

 Its time period was between
200 BCE to 500 BCE. That was
the era of Gupta and Mauryan.
This was the time period when
three religions named as
Hinduism, Buddhism and
Jainism they were getting into a
form and they were creating
their new traditions, during that
era yoga started to emerge.

 During that time period there
were many changes and new
things were added to the yoga,
new methods and practices
were added into the textual form
to be preserved for later
generations. During that era
there were some of main

developments in the favour of yoga those are as Visuddhimagga, the Yoga-Yājñavalkya, the Yoga Sūtras of Patañjali and the Yogācārabhūmi-Śāstra.

Yoga sutra of pantanjali is know as to be the first and the best expression of the brahmanical yoga it was between 325 to 425 BCE. Some of the scholars and experts believe that both of the sutras and the commentary were included in that one.

In some citations there is also some references to that the yoga sutras are taken from the Sramana traditions of Jainism and Buddhism. Also it is possible that Brahman will attempt to adopt this yoga from the traditions of Sramana. There are also a lot of similar concepts in the ancient samkhya, yoga and Buddhist school of thoughts, Abhidharma.

 Also yoga sutras carry the concept of the altered state of the awareness, and the Buddhism concept about the yoga is that it is not for self and not even for the soul and yoga is physical and genuine like samkhya. They believe that so because their religion told them that everyone on the earth has a soule and self.

During this stage of pre-classical yoga, yoga was considered to be something like mishmash of a lot of ideas, techniques, beliefs and the practices. Those usually conflicted to each other and made a contradiction

between all of those concepts.
So the classical stage can be
said as the stage defined by the
Pantanjali sutras of the yoga.
The other name for classical
yoga is RAJA YOGA which was
written in second century. It
defined the practices of the yoga
into 8 different paths. These
steps are the stairs toward the
enlightenment or Samadhi. It is
often consider to be the father of
yoga and still after so many
changes it has a great influence
on the modern yoga and that
influence is great.

Post classic Yoga

Middle age, another
name for this age of
yoga is called post
classical Yoga. During

this age there were many new developments. Many new traditions developed in yoga. The most common know yoga Hatha yoga started in this era. It was the centre point between the classical yoga and the modern world yoga. This was the line from where we started to develop modern yoga. This modern yoga consists of the concept of relief of body, mind and the spirit.

Hatha Yoga

The earliest references to hatha yoga are from Buddhist texts dating back to the eighth century. The first definition of hatha yoga

is found in the 11th
Buddhist text
Vimalaprabha, which
describes it in relation to
the central station, bindu
etc. Hatha yoga
incorporates the
elements of Patanjali's
Yoga Sutras through
exercise and exercise. It
shows the development
of asanas (plural) in the
fully 'used' full body now
widely used and, with its
many modern variations,
the style many people
associate with the word
yoga today.

Sikhism

Various yogic groups
were prominent in the
Punjab in the 15th and
16th centuries, when
Sikhism was relatively
young. The naming of

Gugu Nanak, the founder of Sikhism, describes her many conversations with Jogis, a Hindu community practicing yoga. Gugu Nanak rejected Hatha Yoga-related hardships, customs and traditions. He developed the method of Shahaja yoga or Nama yoga (instead of meditating on the word).

Bhakti Movement

The Bhakti movement was a development in medieval Hinduism that promoted the idea that God is a Person (or "the Supreme Being"). The movement was started by the Alvars of South India in the 6th to 9th centuries, and it began to gain power throughout India in the 12th and 15th centuries. Shaiva and Vaishnava Bhakti combined traditions of Yoga Sutras, as an active meditation exercise, are devoted. The Bhagavad Purana describes a practice of yoga called viraha (separately) Bhakti. Viraha bhakti emphasizes one focus on Khishna.

Hindus Tantra

Tantra is a variant of the esoteric culture that originated in India before the 5th century CE According to George Samuel, "Tantra" is a controversial term, but it can be regarded as a school of practice from the most complete form in Buddhist and Hindu literature by the 10th century CE Tantric yoga developed sophisticated perceptions that involve meditation in the body as a universal microcosm. They include the use of mantras, pranayama, and the subtleties of the body, including nadis and cakras. These teachings on cakras and Kundalini will be among the latest forms of Indian Yoga.

Throughout history, some Tantra school ideas influenced Hindu, Bon, Buddhist, and Jain cultures. Aspects of Tantric yoga practices were adopted and influenced by state practices in the ancient Buddhist and Hindu kingdoms of East and

Southeast Asia. Toward the end of the first millennium, hatha yoga emerged in tantra.

Vajrayana and Tibetan Buddhism

Tantric Buddhism and Tantrayāna are also known as Vajrayana. Its writings were compiled from the seventh century, and the Tibetan translation was completed in the eighth century CE. These texts of tantra yoga were a major source of Buddhist knowledge introduced into Tibet. They were later translated into Chinese and other Asian languages, helping to spread the ideas of Tantric Buddhism. The Buddhist text Hevajra Tantra and Caryāgiti introduced the stages of the chakras. Yoga is an important practice in Tantric Buddhism.

Tantra yoga practices include asanas and breathing exercises. Nyingma tradition uses Yantra yoga (Tib. "Trul khor"): a discipline that includes the practice of breathing (or pranayama), meditation, and other exercises. According to Nyingma tradition, the method of meditation is divided into additional categories, such as Kriya yoga, Upa yoga, Yoga yana, Mahā yoga, Anu yoga and Ati yoga.

Modern Yoga

Since the 19th century, proponents of yoga have modernized yoga through creative translation and settlement processes in response to the ever-increasing increase in capitalism and the colonial and industrial efforts and subsequent international processes. Although modern-day yoga spread throughout the world in the 19th century, its early history was marked by conflicting, superior, or contradictory practices that contradicted common practices and was despised or rejected by many, who often regarded it as the corruption of true yoga or as unacceptable importation. Another, the distinction between the dimensions of meditation, philosophy and morality of yoga, associated with ancient yoga or raja ("royal") yoga, and the physical techniques associated with hatha yoga influence the early form of modern and social yoga .

 After the start of British colonial rule in India, nobles from the United States, Europe, and India dismantled Indian hatha yoga programs in what was considered extremist, violent, and anti-social behaviour. The British colonists and Christian missionaries as well as those Indian dignitaries who were sympathetic to any or both cause the thinking of the Indians to practice hatha yoga as a backlash and a cruel one. Much of this rejection was fuelled by widespread theories about hatha yoga. First, body-wrapping skills in what was considered unusual were associated with the skills of European and North American opponents, so hatha yoga was reduced to Indian crass entertainment. The power of presumed siddhis or the magic of some Hatha yoga practitioners has led to their association of hatha yoga and occult practices. At third Mass distribution texts in certified colonial yoga and Orientalise hatha yoga texts as mysterious, mysterious, uncivilized, and threatening the modern era and the mind.

Revolution of yoga

Representatives of yoga in the 19th and early 20th centuries in Europe and the United States also suffered severe criticism and insistence on their participation in physical yoga. This was a time of religious controversy because of modern analysis that challenged orthodox views. For example, Darwin's theory of evolution was questionable in Orthodoxy. While some major denominations and new religious organizations have responded to such modern challenges by combining elements of various worldviews, sometimes including modern science, others respond with strong religious convictions. Many social and political influences incorporate ecclesiastical values into applying unorthodox oppression of ideologies and practices. The famous efforts of the Postal Inspector Anthony Comstock (1844-1915) serve as an example for the United States.

Consider the life of Ida C. Craddock (1857-1902), an American yoga lawyer who stirred up anger from Comstock and others. Craddock founded the Yoga Church in 1899. He reconstructed the magnitude of the tantric mystico-erotic of hatha yoga into a program by increasing sexual pleasure in a homosexual marriage, and he viewed God as the third partner in a sexual marriage in marriage. In 1902, after being found guilty of defamation in New York, Craddock spent three difficult months in prison. Another government case threatened the prison term. Craddock responded by taking his own life to kill a free woman.

Pierre Bernard (1876-1955)
was another revolutionary yoga
advocate of the 19th century.
His students will continue to
teach yoga until the second half
of the 20th century. Bernard had
a life-affirming vision of yoga
that included modern methods
of yoga - as described below,
this form of yoga was influenced
by modern body culture -
tantra's erotico- mysticism, and
social behaviour based on his
no dualist philosophy. Unlike
many of his modern yoga era in
the United States, including
Indian yoga gurus, which spread
modern yoga translations,
ingenuity and meditation,
Bernard decided on yoga as a
hobby. Therefore, because of
the royal dictatorships that
governed the nation, he had to
keep most of his teachings
secret. Even so, the authorities,

the media, and the Christian clergy made every effort to dissuade Bernard from teaching yoga. For years, he and his students lost their homes and moved to London, where the British authorities deported one of his students who was trying to find students.

Calcutta British Supreme Court Judge Sir John Woodruff (1865–1936) was another modern yoga lawyer who kept most of his work in the mystery of yoga. He read tantric texts, possibly translated by his Bengali friend and pundit, Atul Behari Ghose (1864– 193) , and under the pen of Arthur Avalon, who, in addition to keeping his real name secret, may have represented both Woodruff and

Gose, were published extensively on hatha yoga and tantra. The texts include the Power of the Serpent: The Mysteries of Tantric and Shaktic Yoga (1919), which will be part of the cultural literature list. Further evidence of how hatha yoga was linked to negative ideas in popular Euro-American thought is tied to British magical tantric experiment Aleister Crowley (1875-1947). As a result of such experiments, hatha yoga was associated with the occult in sex.

Others wanted to save yoga from popular opinion and instead promote it as a philosophy, meditation, or morality. They reflect a common tendency in the religious landscape of the 19th and early 20th centuries. As mentioned above, this was a time of religious upheaval for the modern world, leading to the emergence of new environmental, philosophical, and social movements. Transcendentalism, Theosophy, New Thought, Christian Science, and the Vedanta Society and Indian reform organizations, including Brahmo Samaj and the Ramakrishna Mission, were among the many.

In some references the Yoga was adopted by an educated western society in the middle of the 19th century and other subjects of Indian philosophy. In the context of this growing interest, N. C. Paul published his book Treatise on Yoga Philosophy in 1851.

 The first Hindu teacher to actively promote and disseminate the properties of yoga, in addition to asanas, to western audiences, Swami Vivekananda, visited Europe and the United States in the 1890's. The acceptance of Swami Vivekananda was built on the interest of scholars, especially the New England Transcendentalists, among them Ralph Waldo Emerson (1803-1882), who used Roman Romanism and scholars and who had interests (at various levels) in Indian affairs.

 Theosophists including Madame Blavatsky also played a major role in Western society's view of Yoga. The current esoteric ideas of the late 19th century provided another basis for the acceptance of Vedanta and Yoga in its view and the interdisciplinary interaction between the spiritual and the physical. The adoption of Yoga and Vedanta thus merged with each other and the tide (especially based on Neoplatonism) of religious and philosophical reform and transformation throughout the 19th and early 20th centuries. Mircea Eliade has brought something new to the acceptance of Yoga by emphasizing Tantric Yoga in her seminar book: Yoga: Immortality and Freedom. With the introduction of the Tantra culture and the philosophy of Yoga, the "transcendent" conception to be adopted by Yogic practice was removed from the encounter with the "transcendent" ("Atman-Brahman" in Advaitic theory) in the mind itself.

Today, yoga is a major part of a popular culture in urban areas around the world. The postural practice commonly associated with yoga came to prominence in the late 20th century. First, freedom of movement allowed consumers to travel to other parts of the world and receive goods that were different from those of the businessman as well - women, craftsmen, and educators who converted people to spread their teachings or objects outside their residences or regions. Strict immigration restrictions from India to the United States and parts of

Europe were lifted during the 1960's. Second, disillusionment with established religious institutions was widespread as many urban dwellers felt threatened by the prevailing social conditions as a result of globalization and other social ills. Spiritual educators entered the spiritual competitive market with what they considered to be solutions to the extreme problems and turmoil in modern life. They also provided group recognition to people who had been abandoned and the "witchcraft of the world" or "renewal of the world" through their divinity and miracles. Many of them were modern yoga gurus.

Many 20th-century advances have led to the expansion of yoga. Yoga has received much attention from the media, and books on the subject have decided that yoga as one of the most important forms of self-improvement, a goal based on the Protestant concept of individual salvation, which can be combined with other ideas and practices. Indian gurus and European and North American yoga advocates began to rebuild modern yoga in ways that included the world by offering benefits derived from certain nationalities and mysteries of India and instead demonstrated great aspirations for self-improvement. Moreover, instead to rely on the transmission of yoga through traditional practice guru-student relationships, often in a remote ashram state, gurus began to market yoga to a wider audience

Many of the latest widely marketed yoga programs can be labelled as modern stereological yoga, not post-yoga. These programs, unlike popular postural yoga programs, emphasize traditional commitment to greater values and maintain strong organizational structures and doctrinal commitment.

Selvarajan Yesudian (1916-1998) was one of the first Indian yoga advocates in the use of a large market after India. Born in Madras, Yesudian went to Europe in 1936 to study medicine. He met a mysterious Hungarian theologian, Elisabeth Haich (1897-1994), and they wrote the highly successful

Hungarian language book Sport és Jóga (Sport and Yoga) (1941). The book contained photographs of a worthy Yesudian man who performed his posture, breathing exercises and meditation.

Sivananda's recruitment of students from all over the world made Rishikesh a major centre for practicing postural yoga. Yoga was a simple and universal practice, according to Sivananda's, which did not require a physician to abandon a racial, philosophical, or religious commitment. Instead, yoga was intended for anyone who was interested in improving physical and mental health through physical activity. Sogaananda's invention of yoga reached its climax in 1959 with her English book, Yogic Home Exercises: Easy Course of Physical Culture for Modern Men and Women.

One of Sivananda's students in Germany, Boris Sacharow (1899-1959), who had never actually been to Rishikesh, became a student with English-language brochures. In 1947, Sivananda gave him the name yogi raj, or "yoga master." With this honorary title that serves to validate his practice of yoga, Sacharow opened the first yoga school in Germany. One of Sivananda's students, Vishnudevananda (1927-1993), founded the International Sivananda Yoga Vedanta and ashram centres around the country and Sivananda Yoga Teachers' Training Course, which operates to control Sivananda Yoga to this day.

Some of Krishnamacharya's students became yoga entrepreneurs in the background, bringing back yoga to clients across India. Indra Devi (1899-2002) taught back yoga in China and the United States after studying yoga with Krishnamacharya in Mysore. She was originally from Riga, Latvia (formerly Livonia), but ended up in Hollywood, California, where her clients included celebrities, such as Gloria Swanson.

Flourishing the Yoga into the World

Even though Sivananda died in 1963, many of his students succeeded in expanding body-based yoga during this period. Most importantly, Chidananda Sarasvati (1916-2008), who became president of the Divine Life Society after Sivananda's death in 1963, travelled around the world teaching postural yoga and attracting students. Her students included Lilias Folan, who would become famous for teaching postural yoga on American television. However, even before Folan's debut on television, Richard Hittleman's Roga for Health had been featured on various television stations throughout the United States in 1970, and in 1971 it was shown on British television. Eleven years after Hittleman's started Yoga for Health in 1961, 1972, Folan played the first role

Lilias, Yoga, and you! The show started airing on Pincin's PBS station but within a year it was on many PBS stations across the country.

Types of YOGA

There are various methods to perform yoga. Some of those methods are as following.

1. **Buddhist yoga**

2. **Jain yoga**

3. **Tantric yoga**

4. **Hatha yoga**

5. **Laya Yoga and Kundalini yoga**

Buddhist yoga

Buddhist yoga incorporates a variety of techniques that aim to enhance the beauty or essential qualities known as the 37 resurrection aids. The main purpose of Buddhist yoga is bodhi (resurrection) or nirvana (abstinence), traditionally seen as the end of eternal suffering (dukkha) and rebirth. Buddhist texts use many words of spiritual praxis other than yoga, such as bhāvanā ("progress")

and jhāna / dhyāna.

Among the early Buddhists, various forms of yoga were taught, including:

Four dhyāna (four meditation or mental absorption),

Four satipatthatas (foundations

or centres of thought),

Napanasati (spiritual thinking),

Four invisible dwellings (unusual attitude),

Brahmavihārās (divine abodes).

Anussati (thoughts, memories)

This meditation has been regarded as the support of other eight-track paths, such as behavioral practice, right-handed effort, mental self-control, and positive perception. Two mental attributes are important in the practice of yoga in Buddhism, samatha (calmness, stability) and vipassanā (understanding, clear vision). Samatha is a quality of mind stable, relaxed and calm. It is also associated with samadhi (mental integration, concentration) and dhyana (a state of meditation sucking).

Vipassanā is present; the kind of understanding or understanding that goes into the true nature of things. It is also described as "seeing things as they really

are" (yathābhūtaṃ darśanam).

The real nature of things is explained and explained in various ways, but the most important and unique feature of ancient Buddhism is the understanding of all things (dhammas) such the essence of the nature, the doctrine called it

Śūnyatā (the emptiness). This

is in stark contrast to many other Indian cultures, whose intentions are based on the thought of each soul (atman, jiva, pulusha) or the consciousness of all (Brahman). Vipassanā also requires an understanding of suffering or dukkha (and thus four noble truths), impermanence (anicca) and dependence.

 Recent developments in various Buddhist traditions led to new developments in yoga. The Theravada School, while still in its infancy, developed new ideas for meditation and yogic phenomenology in their recent works, the most influential being the Visuddhimagga. The Indic teachings of Mahayana Buddhism can be seen in powerful writings such as the Yogācārabhūmi-Śāstra (compiled about 4th century). Mahayana meditation practices have also developed and embraced new yogic practices, such as the use of mantra and dharan, pure world methods aimed at rebirth in the pure world or Buddha field, and visual methods. Chinese Buddhism improved its methods, such as the Chan practice of Koan and Hua Tou. Similarly, Tantric Buddhism (also Mantrayana, Vajrayana) developed and adopted tantric methods, which remain the basis of the Tibetan Buddhist yogic systems, including the six yogas of Naropa, Kalacakra, Mahamudra and Dzogchen.

Jain Yoga

Jain yoga was a practice centred on Jainism. It is based on the strict code of nonviolence, almsgiving the practice of the austerities like fasting, and yogic practices. Jain yoga aims to liberate and purify the self or soul from the forces of karma, keeping all souls bound in the cycle of migration. Like Yoga and Sankhya, Jainism believes in the multiplicity of isolated souls bound by their karma. It is only with the reduction of karmic infestation and the exhaustion of accumulated karma that the soul can be cleansed and released, at which point one becomes an omniscient person who attains "complete knowledge" (kevala jnana).

The first practice of Jain yoga is divided into many types, includes the meditation

(dhyāna), the abstinence

(kāyotsarga), the meditation

(anuprekṣā), and the meditation (bhāvanā). Other early sources of Jain yoga are Uttarādhyayana sūtra, śvaśyaka sūtra, Sthananga Sutra (c. 2nd century BCE). Recent works include the Vundasunda aṇuvekkhā of the Kundakunda ("The Twelve Thought", c. First century BCE to 1st century CE), the Yogaducisamuccya of Haribhadra (8th century) and the Yogaśāstra of Hemachandra (12th century)). The Hindu influences was embraced later by the Jain yoga, some of the ideas like Patanjali yoga and later Tantric yoga (Hemachandra practices and Haribhadra). They developed a developing way of freedom through the yoga, which defines many levels of the beauty called gunasthanas.

 In modern times, new forms of Jain meditation have also been developed.

Tantric Yoga

Samuel says Tantrism is a contradictory concept. This Tantra yoga is being described as the Samuel, which is being practice by the tantric between the 9th and 10th century in the Hindu and the Buddhist scripts named as Shakti and Saiva, including yogic practices with numerous deities depicting geometric figures and drawings, particularly aggressive male deities. Women, stage-related rituals, extensive use of chakras and mantras, and sexual techniques, all aimed at helping a person's health, the longevity and the freedom.

Hatha Yoga

Hatha yoga, also called hatha vidyā, is a form of yoga that focuses on the exercise of physical and mental strength and posture primarily described in three Hindu texts:

Hatha Yoga Pradipika, Svātmārāma (15th century)

Shiva Samhita, unknown author (1500 or late 17th century)

Gheranda Samhita by Gheranda (late 17th century)

Many scholars can include Goraksha Samhita by the 11th-century Gorakshanath on this list. Gorakshanath is widely regarded as responsible for increasing hatha yoga as we know it today. Other hatha yoga texts include

Haṭhābhyāsapaddhati, Hatha

Ratnavali, Yoga Pradīpikā, and

Sritattvanidhi.

Vajrayana Buddhism, founded by Indian Mahasiddhas, has a series of asanas and pranayama, such as tummo

(Sanskrit caṇḍālī) and trul khor

similar to hatha yoga.

Laya Yoga and Kundalini yoga

These two yogas named as the Laya and the Kundalini yoga are closely related to the Hatha yoga but are often presented as independent methods.

According to the Georg Feuerstein, the Laya yoga (dissolving or combining yoga) "makes meditation the focus of it. Laya-yogin seeks to transcend all traces of memory and sensory experience by removing the microcosm, mind, Self Consciousness." There are various types and techniques of Laya yoga, including listening to the "inner sound" (nada), performing various madras like as Khechari mudra and

Shambhavi mudra and the techniques aimed at the awakening spiritual energy into the body (Kundalini).

The practice of the rejuvenating the body is sometimes called Kundalini yoga. It is based on the Indian concept of a hidden body and uses various breathing techniques body techniques to awaken the energy known as Kundalini (combined) or Shakti. The most common method of teaching this technique is to awaken a Kundalini that lives in the lower chamber of the chakra and lead it through the middle channel to meet the full potential of the highest chakra (above the head).

What is chronic pain?

Chronic pain is a major source of suffering also called **persistent pain** that carries on for longer than 12 weeks even if you do treatments or medications. Most of the patients gets back to their usual life after pain following the operation or let say injury. But sometimes this pain can remain for longer time period or occur without any injury or operation.

In 1900s physicians became to consider the chronic pain before that the only pain which was consider by any doctor or physician was the acute pain like the pain of any injury or like the pain of surgery. That was all consider to be a pain and if somebody would ask any doctor about the chronic pain they thought that it was some side effect of medicines or the patients is taking drugs. People were not aware of that condition and the patients suffered a lot from that. There was no proper knowledge or education related to chronic pain. Those patients who do not want to use the drugs or do not have proper access turned towards the neurosurgery or they were asked to get psychotherapy form someone.

The chronic pain obviously affects the body of a person but it also leaves a very strong effect on the brain of the people, also it affects relationships and emotions of a person. As due to this continuous pain, people's behaviour change and they become like being irritated form everybody and they could not

get relief from this pain due to
that there mental health is also
effected which causes in the
loss of relationships in their life.
Due to that continuous pain they
could not concentrate on the
work and it brought them the
stress which is a clear health
issue. When mind is not in
peace then how can the person
lives in peace.

   More than 25 percent of the
people of the world going
through chronic pain start to
face the condition called chronic
pain syndrome.

Chronic Pain Syndromes (CPS)

   So the basic cause of chronic
pain syndromes is that when we
have chronic pain and we
cannot get rid of it and with the
passage of the time like 3 to 6

months, that continuous pain effect our mental health causes stress, anxiety and depression which also cause the disturbance in their daily life. This condition is the worst in the case of the chronic pain.

To treat a patient having chronic pain syndromes is hard to treat.

So basically it starts with the chronic pain. That chronic pain could be any type of pain, like the pain of joint problem, pain of back, headaches, muscle strain, repetitive stress of injuries, broken bones, cancer, Fibromyalgia, nerve damage or many other serious pains, which stays for longer time.

So the chronic pain syndrome (CPS) is the condition of both mentally disturbance and physically disease. This type of pain affects both male and females regard less the limit of age. But it is the most common pain in women. People suffering through this pain, their behaviour change and even after the relief they keep their bad behaviour towards other which cause the broke in relations.

To examine chronic pain syndrome there are several symptoms. Some of those are written here from them you can examine yourself and do the proper treatment.

As we know that these continuous pains lead many more diseases therefore the most appropriate method to fight the chronic pain is YOGA. Yoga helps us to fight this chronic pain and get relief. It is certain that in this era there are many treatments but as we have already discussed about the negligence of professionals who are sitting there to only make money, they will do more harm to you rather than to treat you. Recently I came to know about a patient who told me his story that he was facing pain in his lower back. When he went to see the doctor, doctor could not locate the proper cause of pain and advice me of some kind of surgery. After going through the surgery I am still facing the same pain and when I went back to that doctor he told me that it is only my perception. And after going through many tests from many experts they could not find the cause of chronic pain. As from the above incident it is not wise to visit someone who does not have proper knowledge. To avoid such incidents it is mandatory to have basic knowledge about the chronic pain and yoga is the best self treatment. Yoga helps you to get relief physically and emotionally.

Cause of chronic pain

Generally the cause of chronic pain has been not yet discovered properly due to less attention towards this disease. If we see it scientifically then the actual cause of the pain is that all the nerves are connected in the body. But here we are talking about the reasons which cause those nerves to activate so the chronic pain is usually caused by injury an initial injury like back sprain or the pulled muscle. Some doctors believe that the chronic pain is cause by the damage of the nerves, it causes the pain for long lasting time and it makes pain more severe. So in these cases of nerves damage the issue of pain will not be resolved by treating the injury.

People do however experience chronic pain without the injury or without having any wound. This is the most terrifying cause of chronic pain, which is without having any injury or wound. These chronic pains may sometimes cause from the different health conditions such as

Chronic fatigue syndrome: This condition is caused by the in many cases due to stress. Many experts says it is not possible to understand the cause of this pain, but this pain is long lasting that is why it is consider to be the symbol of stress and depression. There is no testing for the identification of this pain.

Endometriosis: It can affect women of any age and it is cause by similar tissues to the lining of womb grow in other places. It is a very long lasting pain which will definitely affect the life of women, due to its long lasting impact it is the cause of chronic pain in the patient.

Fibromyalgia: It is a very common pain and very long lasting impacts are left behind on the health of patient. It is a very widespread emotion of pain; it is a very long lasting pain round about al least 3 months. Its tender points are located in chest, neck, hips, in the elbows, knees, shoulders and in short all over the main joints of a human body. When people leave this untreated and pay no attention it causes the chronic pain in the body which is a very alarming condition. Which causes stress and mode disorders in the patients and in some cases even much more worst.

Inflammatory bowel disease: In this condition people experience pain of two or more conditions but basically it is consider being the group of two conditions. Those two conditions are Crohn's disease and ulcerative colitis. It causes the chronic pain if it is not treated on time. The mental state of the person experiencing this condition also affects a lot.

Interstitial cystitis: Its absolute reason is unknown. If it is left without treatment then it can have a very long term affects on the life of the patient. It leads towards the chronic pain and loss of mental peace. Also people going through this condition, people face pain and problem in peeing. It is very irritating and become the cause of mental and physical health problems..

Temporomandibular joint dysfunction (TMJ): it is the term used for the pain of jaw muscles, those muscles which moves jaw and this pain does directly feels like we are having pain in skull. As those joints are directly connected to the skull and from that our whole body remains at stress as we cannot avoid the pain here and the most irritating pin is this and it causes the loss of emotions and relationships. As we are not at peace then our nature will gradually becomes more intense and will cause in the disorder of routine. Id this pain continues for long time then it causes the pain of chronic pain.

As we can see the mostly small problems grow into larger ones and then cause the unpleasant life order. That is why it is mandatory to keep good care our health and also the mental peace.

Types of chronic pain

Everybody experience occasional pains, and in origin

sudden pain is a reaction of
nervous system which help us to
determines that there is some
kind of injury, and these nervous
signals our brain and in the
reaction to these nervous
signals our brain automatically
reacts and we try to cover that
part, where injury had happened
our will do in our best way to
handle that injury or that pain.
So when we are facing chronic
pain then our nervous system
continuously send the signals to
our brain, and in the result of
those nervous signals we feel a
non stop pain. That non stop
pain is called chronic pain.
These signals created by the
nervous they travel from the part
where they sense some injury or
anything similar to that, causing
the pain, and first they went to
spinal cord and then from over
there to our brain. Then we feel

pain after receiving those signals.

As with the passage of time the injury heals and the pain become less severe and our body become relaxed. So in the case of chronic pain our brain continuously receive signals from our injured area which has been healed properly and this chronic pain last more than months. It will completely change your life and will affect your daily life very seriously. Due to that we do face a lot of challenges daily and our mobility gets limited and also the flexibility and strength.

Some of the most common types of chronic pain include:

- **Chronic Daily Headache**

- **Post Surgical pain**

- **Post-trauma pain**

- **Lower back pain**

- **Cancer pain**

- **Arthritis pain**

- **Neurogenic pain (pain caused by nerve damage)**

- **Psychogenic pain (pain that isn't caused by disease, injury, or nerve damage)**

Chronic Daily Headache:

As this daily life routine is so busy for everyone therefore we can face sometime headache. It is basically due to tiredness or due to some blood pressure issues. Many people in this world do have headaches form a specific piece of time to time.

That headache is not the cause
of worry that is normal like I said
due to tiredness or blood
pressure issues. There is a
condition when you feel pain for
more than weeks in your head;
in that situation that pain is not
normal that is the symptom of
chronic daily headache.

Chronic daily headache has
many kind of subtypes, and it
includes that how often a
headache remains and how long
does it remains, let say that
what is the how often it occurs
and how long it remains.

Due to this continuous chronic
daily headache person becomes

more irritating and is the most worst headache condition.

Two types are there for the chronic daily headache, one of these is called long-lasting chronic headache and the other one is called short-lasting daily headache. As we can assume from the names of these two types of chronic daily headache long-lasting chronic daily headache last for more time and its time period is more than 4 to 5 hours a day.

The long-lasting chronic daily headache includes:

- **Daily Static headache**

- **Hemicranias continua**

- **Chronic migraine**

- **Chronic tension-type headache**

Daily Static headache:

This condition is for those patients who are already having some serious issues and have some history of headache. In this situation patients feel headache on the both side of the head. When someone is going through this pain he or she will feel like something is pressing or pushing and the head is being tightened. And it will become consistent within three to four days of first headache. It causes the mild to moderate pain. It seems similar

to the chronic tension type pain
or headache.

Hemicranias continua:

The person who is facing this
type of headache is often
consider to be having the pain
on one side of head, it is
continuous pain and there is no
free time. Means that the patient
will continuously feel the pain
and it will never stop even for a
moment. From this condition
you can understand that how
much severe condition is this for
a person. It also cause
moderate pain with spikes of
severe headache. It becomes
more severe with the passage of
time that is another moment for
consideration that it can take

you to the ultimate level of
stress.

The symptoms for more clarity
are having redness in the eye
on the effected side. People
facing this pandemic feel nasal
congestion or runny nose. Also
there is pupil narrowing and
drooping eyelid in the symptoms
of this pain.

Chronic migraine:

This situation is related to
the people who have some
history of episodic
migraines. It is same as
like Hemicranias with some
less severe condition. It is
also same to be on one
side of head, it has
pulsating and throbbing
sensation. It cause

moderate to severe
condition pain. In the result
of this patient starts to
vomiting or nausea or in
some cases both
conditions applies. People
with this headache are very
sensitive to light and
sound. They do not want
any noise near them
otherwise it hurts them a
lot.

**Chronic tension-type
headache**

It causes both sides of the head
to be in pain also it causes the
mild to moderate the headache,
in this pain is like pressing but
not like pulsating.

Causes

Although there could be many
causes to the severe chronic

daily headache, those causes are not very well known or let say considered. Some of those conditions which cause this chronic daily headache are as following.

First of all the most common cause is the problems with blood vessels in the brain and around the brain also the inflammation, you can also count the stroke. Secondly the other cause which could be possibly the root to the chronic daily headache is infections for example meningitis. It can cause the continuous pain in the head.

After that the blood pressure that is high or low I mean in the most low blood pressure and in the most high blood pressure condition these pain can be developed. Despite all of that another serious condition could be brain tumor. That is the most dangerous condition for the life of a patient. Another cause for the chronic daily headache is traumatic brain injury in the result of some accident or like that being hit on the head.

Medication overuse headache:

Usually this type of headache happens due to tension and migraine type and due to that reason they take medicines, pain killers in more quantity than needed. Due to over dose of medicines they face this type of chronic daily headache. So be careful while taking medicine for headache for too long that will affect the whole system and will give you more severe condition.

Some basic factors attached with developing chronic daily headache are as following.

Factors associated with developing frequent headaches include:

- Obesity

- Snoring

- Female sex

- Depression

- Anxiety

- Sleep Disorder

- Overdose of caffeine

- Overdose of headache medication

- Many other chronic pain conditions

It is defined as the pain which lasts more than 12 weeks or lest say which last more than 3 to 6 months. After going through this pain person who is facing can have some serious impacts like causing aching sensation or a burning at the place where it was affected. It could be in both possible situations like steady pain or intermittence, feeling or be at peace without any reason. Any part of the person's body can be affected by this chronic pain wich may last for more than usual time period. So if you are having chronic daily headache, then it is more in advance that you might as well have the sleep disorder, anxiety, depression, physical issues and as well as other psychological issues in addition.

Post Surgical pain

In many cases after the surgery patients feels the pain which last for a very longer period. That pain is called chronic post surgical pain in short CPSP. It lasts longer than the normal healing process and it is an unwanted worst event after any surgery. It was first discovered in 1999 by Macrae and Davies. After some time more research on it prove it to be the most critical pain condition which lasts for at least two months.

It can lead the patients towards to a severe condition, including the conditions of functional limitation and psychological trauma.

Although there are many medications for the relief but the most affective suggested by any expert to do exercise and yoga is the best fit in all of them to heal you and your soul and help you to return to your normal life after the severe condition of the Chronic post surgical pain.

Post-trauma pain

Any serious physical injury is called "physical trauma." It is not uncommon for a patient to experience persistent, severe pain for no apparent reason after the initial injury. Post-traumatic pain is any pain that occurs after the healing of an injury from physical trauma.

There are two main types of physical abuse:

Blunt force trauma: in which an object or force strikes the body with sufficient force to cause a collision, a deep cut, or a broken bone.

Trauma that penetrates: when an object pierces the skin and forms an open wound.

Other common types of traumatic injuries include traumatic brain injury, spinal injuries, spinal fractures, traumatic amputations, facial trauma, acoustic trauma, bruising injuries, fractures and broken bones.

Cause for Post trauma Chronic pain

Post-traumatic stress after traumatic injury is common. In many cases, chronic pain is the result of emotional trauma (causalgia or mimocausalgia) caused by trauma. Vascular injuries are often the cause of ongoing pain even after treatment has ended.

No injury is too minor to cause post-traumatic stress disorder. Even the spine can cause post-traumatic stress disorder. In fact, this nerve does not need to be damaged to cause pain. Sometimes, muscle pressure due to injury is enough to cause pain that can range from mild to severe discomfort.

Doctors do not fully understand why some injuries cause chronic pain; however, it is believed that

it may be a mistaken link
between the central and
peripheral nervous systems, and
an improper inflammatory
response.

For example, arthritis,
inflammation of the joints, can
be the cause of post-traumatic
arthritis pain. Post-traumatic
arthritis (cartilage dislocation) is
a common form of osteoarthritis
that can occur after any type of
physical injury to the joint.

Symptoms

After a traumatic injury, some

discomfort is expected. The pain can be mild and intense. Over time, the symptoms of pain may change and will vary from patient to patient.

Often, pain, swelling, redness, noticeable changes in skin temperature, and hypersensitivity (especially cold and touch) are the first symptoms of post-traumatic stress disorder. Patients often describe post-traumatic pain as "burning," "unpleasant itching," or "numbness," which are symptoms similar to other forms of nerve pain such as sores.

Some of the most common

symptoms of post trauma
chronic pain are as following:

1. Some of the symptoms
   for the post traumatic
   disorder are mentioned
   as follow

2. Persistent burning or
   throbbing pain: usually in
   the arm, hand, leg, or
   foot.

3. Changes in skin
   temperature: The skin
   may appear sweaty and
   cold.

4. Changes in skin color:
   The skin may appear

white and have red or
blue spots.

5. Changes in skin
composition: The skin
can become soft and
sensitive when touched.
The skin becomes shiny
and more thin of the
affected part.

6. Change in the hair and
the nail growth.

7. The ability to move the
affected part gradually
decreases with time
passage

8. Joint stiffness, swelling, and injury

9. Muscle dysfunction, weakness, and loss (atrophy).

10. Sensitivity to touch or cold: The area may be very sensitive to touch or cold.

11. Inflammation of the painful area

12. Pain can be exacerbated by emotional distress.

In some patients, the symptoms go away at their own time. For some, chronic pain and dysfunction may persist for months or years.

If not detected and treated early, post-traumatic stress disorder can develop and worsen symptoms, which may include:

Atrophy: The patients often avoid moving an arm or leg because it is painful, or difficult to walk due to stiffness. If part of the body is not moving, the skin, bones, and muscles may begin to shrink and deteriorate.

Contract (muscle stiffness): The patient can experience the strengthening of their muscles.

This can lead to a situation where the hand and fingers, or the foot and toes, get into a position.

Diagnosis

The nervous system has millions of nerves throughout the human body. Post-traumatic stress disorder can be the result of any of these nerves being affected by different types of trauma.

Diagnosis of chronic post-traumatic pain is based primarily on physical examination and medical history of the patient. Unfortunately, no single trial can actually diagnose post-traumatic stress disorder, but there are diagnostic procedures that can provide important clues, such as:

Circulatory sensory blocks: This procedure attempts to prevent the cause of the suspected and chronic pain syndrome to determine which sensor may need to be considered to resolve the symptoms.

Bone scan: A test to find bone change, the radiation device is inserted into a vein to aid in the appearance of bones with a special camera.

Sensory system testing:
These tests look for
disturbances in the sensitive
nervous system (skin
temperature, blood flow) in the
affected and unaffected organs.

X-rays: Loss of minerals in the
bones can appear on X-ray in
the later stages of the disease.

**Magnetic resonance imaging
(MRI):** Images from MRI may
show tissue changes.

Other tests can be used to
measure the amount of sweat
produced by both organs.
Unexplained consequences are
a potential indicator of post-

traumatic stress disorder. A blood test, a measure of erythrocyte sedimentation (ESR), can be performed to rule out diseases with similar symptoms from other causes.

In this conditions of post traumatic stress, patient faces the most painful experience and the mind of that person becomes like dull and dark. That person could not get peace, or the peace of body neither the peace of mind.

Lower back chronic pain

If you have ever had mild pain, you are not alone. This is

becoming the most rising cause to see the doctor by many people in these days. Due to this reason many patients lost their jobs as they could not give time to their job. This back pain could catch the person of any age and any gender.

Back pain can range from mild to severe, lasting longer than sudden, sharp, or shooting pain. It can start suddenly as a result of an accident or lift something heavy, or it can start later as we grow older. Excessive exercise followed by exercise can also cause back pain.

There are two types of back

pain:

Severe back pain: or temporary
pain lasts for a few days to a
few weeks. Most low back pain
is severe. It usually resolves on
its own in a few days of self-care
and there are no job losses left.
In some cases it can take time
and even up to a few months to
heal properly or let say to get rid
of that pain.

Chronic back pain: It is defined
as pain that lasts 12 weeks or
more, whether initial treatment
or the underlying cause of back
pain is treated. About 20 percent
of people affected by low back
pain develop chronic back pain

and persistent symptoms within a year. Even if the pain remains constant, it does not means that it can be easily identified and treated or do have a medical cause. In some cases, treatment effectively relieves chronic back pain, but in other cases the pain persists despite treatment and treatment.

Back structure

To better understand about this pain we need to know more about the structure of back which is describe as following

The lower back - where most back pain is most common -

includes five vertebrae (called L1-L5) in the lumbar region, which support a lot of upper body weight. Intervertebral discs that act as shock absorbers throughout the spinal column to prevent bones as the body moves also called round pads they have some space which is being maintained. Tissue belts known as ducts hold the spinal cord in place, and the muscles attach to the spinal column. Thirty-one nerve pairs are centered in the spine and control body movements and transmit signals from the body to the brain.

Other vertebrate regions are the

uterus (neck), thoracic (upper
back), and sacral and coccygeal
(below the lumbar region).

Cause for back pain

Most painful back pain is
mechanical in nature, meaning
that there is a disruption in the
way the parts of the spine
(spine, muscles, intervertebral
discs, and nerves) meet and
move.

 Some examples of the causes
of low back pain include:

The womb

Bone disorders: such as scoliosis (spinal curvature), Lordosis (excessively exaggerated arch in the lower back), kyphosis (external arch of the spine), and other spinal deformities.

Spine bifida: involves incomplete growth of the spine and / or its protective cover and can cause problems including vertebrae deformities and abnormal sensations and even disability.

Injuries

Sprains (stretched or torn muscles): strains (tears in muscles or tendons), and spasms (sudden contraction of a muscle or group of muscles)

Severe injuries: such as sports, car accidents, or falls that can injure muscles, tendons, or muscles that cause pain, as well as compression of the spine and cause discs to explode or attack.

Changing problems

Intervertebral disc degeneration that occurs when discs of rubber usually age as a normal process of aging and loses their ability to pull.

Spondylosis is a common spinal degeneration associated with normal wear and tear that occurs in joints, discs, and spinal cord as people grows older.

Arthritis or other inflammatory diseases of the spine: including osteoarthritis and rheumatoid arthritis and spondylitis, inflammation of the vertebrae.

Emotional and spinal problems

Spinal compression,

inflammation and / or injury

Sciatica (also called radiculopathy): is caused by something that compresses the sciatic nerve that runs down the hips and down the back of the leg. People with sciatica can feel shocked — or even burn low-level pain associated with pain in one and the same leg and leg.

Spinal stenosis: the spinal column that puts the pressure on the spinal cord and nerves of the body are very narrow.

Spondylolisthesis which occurs when the lower vertebra

of the lower spine slips out of
place compresses the nerves
from the spinal column.

Herniated or fractured discs
can occur when Intervertebral
discs are compressed and
ruptured externally.

Infections involving the
vertebrae, a condition called
osteomyelitis; Intervertebral
discs, called discitis; or
sacroiliac joints that connect the
lower back and pelvis, called
sacroiliitis.

Cauda equina syndrome occurs
when a fractured disc reaches
the spinal cord and compresses

the mass of the lumbar and sacral nerve roots. Permanent nerve damage may occur if the disease is left untreated.

Osteoporosis (continuous degeneration of bones and energy that can lead to painful fractures of the vertebrae)

Non-spinal sources

Kidney stones can cause severe pain in the lower back, usually on one side

Endometriosis (formation of
uterine tissue in areas outside
the uterus)

Fibromyalgia (a chronic pain
disorder that is associated with
increased muscle pain and loss)

Abscesses compress or
destroy the spinal cord or spine
and nerves or outside the spine
elsewhere in the back

Pregnancy (back symptoms are
almost completely gone after
childbirth)

**Risk Factors for Chronic back
pain**

There are many factors due to which we can have a severe back pain, a chronic back pain, and that pain could make our life worst more than any other pain. Some of those risk factors are bellow to help you keep safe from chronic pain.

Anyone can have back pain. Factors that can increase the risk of low back pain include:

Age: The first attack of low back pain occurs most commonly between the ages of 30 and 50, and back pain becomes more common with aging. Bone loss from osteoporosis can lead to fractures, and at the same time, muscle stiffness and tone decrease. Intervertebral discs begin to lose fluid and adapt to age, reducing their ability to protect the vertebrae. The risk of spinal stenosis is also increasing.

Severity level: Back pain is more common in people who are physically unfit. Weak muscles in the back and abdomen may not support the spine properly. All of those people who do daily exercise and make it a routine they face less chances of getting back pain. And the people who do exercise or gym after some time and they do not make it continuous habit they face this experience of back pain in more strength. Studies show that low-impact exercise can help maintain the integrity of intervertebral discs.

Weight gain: Obesity, obesity, or rapid weight gain can put pressure on your back and lead to lower back pain.

Genetics: Other causes of back pain, such as ankylosing spondylitis (a type of arthritis involving the joints of the spine that lead to spinal instability), are genetic.

Job-related factors: Having a job that requires heavy lifting, pushing, or pulling, especially if it involves twisting or twisting the spine, can lead to injuries and back pain. Working at a desk all day can be a source of pain, especially from standing or sitting in a chair without adequate back support.

Mental health: Anxiety and depression can affect how a person focuses on their pain and their perception of its severity. Chronic pain may play a role in the development of such psychological factors. Depression can affect the body in many ways, including causing muscle spasms.

Smoking: It can block the flow of blood and oxygen to the discs, causing them to lose weight faster.

Backpack for children: A backpack full of school books and supplies can pull back and cause muscle fatigue.

Psychological factors: Emotions and depression, stress, and mental well-being can also affect the chances of back pain.

Arthritis pain

Rheumatoid arthritis (RA) is an incurable inflammatory disease. It usually starts in small joints in the hands and feet. RA causes pain, stiffness and swelling. Mobility and flexibility in the affected joints is also being reduced.

As RA progresses, these symptoms can spread to other areas, including:

1. waist

2. shoulders

3. ankles

4. Elbows

5. wrists

6. ankles

Neurogenic pain (pain caused by nerve damage)

Neuropathic is a pain which is many times said as shooting or burning pain. It can go away on its own but is often an incurable disease. Sometimes it never ends and it is difficult, and sometimes it comes and goes. It is usually the result of nerve damage or a dysfunctional nervous system. The impact of nerve damage is a change in the functioning of both nerves in the area of injury and surrounding areas.

Phantom limb syndrome is an example of chronic neuropathic pain in a person. This rare condition occurs when an arm or leg is removed due to illness or injury, but the brain still receives pain messages from the nerves that carried the nerves from that missing leg. These nerves are now very hot and cause pain.

Causes

Categories named as morbidity, injury, infection, and weight loss are considered to be the most common causes of neuropathic pain.

Diseases

Neuropathic pain can be a symptom or problem of several diseases and conditions. Multiple sclerosis, multiple myeloma, and other types of cancer are being included in it.

Not all of the patients experiencing these conditions do experience neuropathic pain, but in some cases it can be a tremendous problem for patients.

 Chronic diabetes can affect the way your nerves work. it is responsible for more than 30 percent of the chronic neuropathic pain cases, according to the Cleveland Clinic.

People with diabetes often experience numbness and numbness, followed by pain, burns and injuries to their joints and joints. Prolonged exposure to alcohol can lead to many problems, including chronic neuropathic pain. Emotional harm to alcohol abuse can have long-lasting and devastating effects.

Trigeminal neuralgia is a painful condition with severe neuropathic pain on one side of the face. It is one of the most common types of neuropathic pain and can occur for no known reason. Finally, cancer treatment can cause neuropathic pain. Chemotherapy and radiation can affect the nervous system and cause unusual pain signals.

Injuries

Damage to muscles, tendons, or joints is a rare cause of neuropathic pain. Similarly, problems with the back or leg, leg, or injury can cause permanent damage to the arteries.

While the injury may heal, the damage to the nervous system may not go away. As a result, you may experience chronic pain for many years after the accident. Injuries or injuries that affect the spine can also cause neuropathic pain, too. Nerve fibers around your spine can be damaged by the compression of spinal cord and Herniated discs.

Infection

Diseases do not usually cause

neuropathic pain. Shingles, caused by the outbreak of chicken pox, can cause several weeks of neuropathic pain in the arteries. Infection with syphilis can also lead to burns, relieving unexplained pain. People with HIV can feel this inexplicable pain.

Loss of organs

A rare form of neuropathic pain called phantom limb syndrome can occur when amputated an arm or a leg. Even if you lose that limb, your brain still thinks they are getting painful signals from a removed body part.

What really happens, though, is that the nerves close to amputation may not function properly and send the wrong signals to your brain.

It does not have any specific cause. But other common causes of neuropathic pain include:

1. Excessive drinking

2. Determination

3. Chemotherapy

4. Diabetes

5. Emotional problems on the face

6. HIV infection or AIDS

7. Multiple myeloma

8. Multiple sclerosis

9. Nerve or spinal compression from herniated discs or arthritis in the spine

10. Swords

11. Spinal surgery

12. Syphilis

13. Thyroid problems

So this is also a chronic pain
condition which can make the
patient's life more worst and the
person going through this would
feel his life like a hell.

Psychogenic pain (pain that
isn't caused by
disease, injury, or
nerve damage)

Psychogenic pain is a term for
pain caused mainly by
psychological factors, such as
depression and anxiety. While
psychogenic pain can be
caused by physical pathology, it
is a real form of chronic pain.
People with depression and

anxiety may report psychogenic pain throughout their body, even for no apparent physical reason.

Psychogenic pain is often more difficult to treat than nociceptive pain or neuropathic pain. Traditional painkillers are designed to treat physical ailments, such as inflammation or nervous disorders. With psychogenic pain, however, there are often no physical causes for diagnosis and treatment. Non-pharmacological therapies, such as TENS and disorders, tend to be more effective in reducing psychogenic pain than traditional painkillers.

Causes

Although this pain is very real to those who experience it, there is no specific test to determine if you have mental pain. This type of pain can have many different psychological factors that can create, exacerbate, or maintain pain:

1. Beliefs

2. Emotions

3. Fear

4. Mental illness such as depression or anxiety

In this condition nerve is sometimes considered to be damage that is why patient is facing pain, but its main concept is related to psychological problems. Its main concern is with the brain.

Yoga and Chronic pain

Yoga is the main source for the spiritual relief, body and the mind relief. As the YOGA does not consists of only some oral words it contains a lot of exercises and the postures that can help you to get relief for any kind of chronic pain. As we know chronic pain is something which cannot be treated by the help of medicines. At that point when there is no use of medicines on the body to give you relief from that severe pain, then the YOGA comes as the leading ray of the light of hope. Yoga treats someone's external and as well as the internal pains.

Here we will teach you some of those exercises which can help you to gain more peaceful life. It will treat your chronic pain which you might have been suffering through, right now. First chapter which you will have to learn is to not visit any doctor or any physician. As we have already discussed that these doctors do not have proper knowledge so they will ask you for unnecessary test or will give you wrong prescription. Even they without knowing the actual cause of disease will ask you for operations or something like that. So it is not wise to visit any doctor if you are having chronic pain.

Yoga is the best solution to every chronic pain, and for generations it has helped patients suffering through this miserable condition of chronic pain. People have experienced the yoga as the medication for chronic pain and after a lot of research it is now being recommended by many doctors to do yoga. Here are some of the yoga techniques which will help you to fight the chronic pain in your life.

Yoga Exercise

If you are suffering from back pain, yoga can be what the doctor prescribed. Yoga is a form of psychotherapy that is often recommended to treat not only back pain but also the accompanying stress. Proper conditions can relax and strengthen your body.

Practicing yoga even for a few minutes a day can help you to become more aware of your body. This will help you to identify where you are holding the conflict and where you have the inequality. You can use this information to bring yourself to balance and understanding.

  Keep reading to learn more about how these conditions can help treat back pain.

  This exercise will help you to be fully able to do backbend stretches and mobilizes the spine of your body. The shoulders, neck and torso also stretches by the help or by practicing the pose which is named as backbend.

  During this process the muscles of our body like triceps, serratus anterior, gluteus ,aximus, erector spinae and rectus abdominis work and these muscles stretches which help to keep the back of the body to be more flexible and it helps to heal the lower back body.

Procedure for the Cat-Cow exercise is as following:

1. First of all sit down on the floor and make a position by getting on all the four. Get on the both hands and the knees, facing the floor.

2. You should be in the position where the knees underneath your hips and the wrist underneath your shoulders.

3. Your weight should be balanced equally between all of the four points of body.

4. Inhale the air as you will look upside and at that point your stomach should drop down in the direction of the floor.

5. When you will exhale the air then at that time tuck your chin into the chest and take your navel in the direction of your spine and raise your spine in the direction of the sky.

6. While doing this movement your body should be maintained.

7. Keep your focus on releasing the tension from your body.

8. Keep doing these steps for at least 1 minute.

Downward-Facing Dog

This yoga exercise can be useful and rejuvenating. This pose helps to get relief from the chronic back pain. It helps to increase the strength in the body and also helps to imbalances.

During this process the muscles of our body like quadriceps, hamstrings, deltoids, aximus, gluteus maximus and triceps work and these muscles stretches which help to keep the back of the body to be more flexible and it helps to heal the chronic back pain in the body.

Procedure for the Cat-Cow exercise is as following:

1. Get on the floor and get in a position of on all fours

2. Your knees should be under the hips and hands should be in alignment under your wrists.

3. Tuck your toes under while pressing into your hands and then lift the knees up.

4. The sitting bones should be in the direction of the ceiling.

5. There should be a slight bend in the knees so it will lengthen the tailbone and your spine.

6. Your heals should be a little bit up from the ground

7. Press into the hands more forcefully and strongly.

8. The weight should be on the both sides and distributed equally. The position of the

shoulders and hips
should be in attention.

9. This chin tucked in a
    little bit and head
    should be in a straight
    line with upper

10. Continue this pose for
    at least 1 minute.

Extended Triangle

This normal posture can help
reduce back pain, sciatica,
and neck pain. It stretches the
spine, waist, and groans, and
strengthens the shoulders,
chest, and legs. It can also
help to get relief from chronic
back pain.

During this process the

muscles of our body like latissimus dorsi, internal oblique, gluteus maximus and medius, muscles, gluteus maximus and quadriceps and these muscles stretches which help to keep the back of the body to be more flexible and it helps to heal the chronic back pain in the body.

To do the yoga pose of this Extended Triangle you will have to do following procedure that will help you to get relief from suffering:

1. From a standstill, walk your feet four feet [4 m] apart.

2. Turn your right toes
    forward, and your left
    toes at an angle.

3. Raise your arms
    straight down with your
    palms facing down.

4. Bend forward and then
    insert your right hinge
    to move forward with
    your arm and body.

5. Bring your hand to
    your leg, yoga block,
    or floor.

6. Extend your left arm
    towards the sky.

7. Look up, forward, or
    down.

8. Continue in this
    position for at least 1
    minute

9. Repeat on the other
   side.

Sphinx Pose

This gentle backbend
strengthens your spine and
buttocks. Stretching your
chest, shoulders and
abdomen. It can also help
reduce stress.

Muscles worked:

1. erector spinae

2. radiant muscles

3. large pectoralis

4. trapezius

5. latissimus dorsi

To do this:

1. Lie on your stomach with your legs open behind you.

2. Combine your lower back muscles, buttocks, and thighs.

3. Bring your elbows under your shoulders with your arms down and your palms facing down.

4. Slowly raise your upper chest and head.

5. Gently lift and flex your lower abdomen to support your back.

6. Be sure to lift your spine and exit with the crown of your head, instead of falling on your lower back.

7. Keep your eye focused as you are completely relaxed in this pose, while at the same time staying active and involved.

8. Keep continuing this position for at least five minutes.

Cobra Pose

This gentle backbend lightens your abdomen, chest and shoulders. Practicing this pose strengthens your spine and can relieve sciatica. It can also help reduce the stress and fatigue that can accompany back pain.

Muscles worked:

1. muscles
2. gluteus maximus
3. deltoids
4. triceps
5. serratus earlier

To do this:

1. While your fingers are facing forward then lie on your stomach and your hands should be under the shoulders.

2. Draw your arms and hold them to your chest. Do not let your elbows slip.

3. Press your hands to raise the head, chest and shoulders slightly.

4. You can lift half, half, or all the way up.

5. Keep a slight bend in your elbows.

6. You can let your head go back to deepen the posture.

7. Release the back of
    your mat on the
    exhale.

8. Rest your head and
    bring the arms to your
    side.

9. Slowly move your hips
    back and forth to
    relieve tension in your
    lower back.

Locust Pose

This gentle backbend can
help relieve low back pain and
fatigue. It strengthens the
back chest, arms and legs.

Muscles worked:

1. trapezius

2. erector spinae

3. gluteus maximus

4. triceps

To do this:

1. Lie on your stomach with your hands close to your chest and your hands up.

2. Touch your big toes together and pull your heels to the side.

3. Put your forehead slightly down.

4. Raise your head, chest, and arms

slowly, halfway, or all
the way up.

5. You can bring your
   hands together and
   put your fingers behind
   your back.

6. To deepen the stand,
   lift your legs.

7. Look forward or
   upward as you raise
   the back of your neck.

8. Continue in this pose
   for at least 1 minute.

9. Take a break before
   pausing again.

Bridge Pose

This is a reversal and a
change that can trigger or
reverse. It stretches the spine
and may relieve back and
head.

Muscles worked:

1. rectus and transverse
    abdominis

2. gluteus muscles

3. erector spinae

4. muscles

To do this:

1. Lie on your back with
    your knees bent and

your heels pulled to
your sitting bones.

2. Relax your arms next
   to your body.

3. Press your feet and
   arms down as you lift
   your tail up.

4. Keep lifting until your
   thighs are aligned on
   the floor.

5. Leave your arms as
   they are, bring the
   palms of your hands
   together with the
   fingers folded under
   your hips, or place
   your hands under your
   hips for support.

6. continue in this style
   for at least 1 minute.

7. Loosen by bending
   your spine back down,
   vertebra by vertebra.

8. Put your knees
   together.

9. Relax and breathe
   deeply into this place.

Half Lord of the Fishes

This cleansing pose
strengthens your spine and
helps relieve back pain.
Stretch your hips, shoulders,
and neck. This posture can
help reduce fatigue and
rejuvenate your internal

organs.

Muscles worked:

1. rhomboids

2. serratus earlier

3. erector spinae

4. large pectoralis

5. psoas

To do this:

1. From where you sit,
    draw your right foot
    closer to your body.

2. Bring your left foot out
    of your leg.

3. Stretch the spine while twisting the body to the left side.

4. Take your left hand down behind your back for support.

5. Move your right arm out of your left thigh, or tie your elbow to your left knee.

6. Try to maintain your buttocks to deepen the twists in your spine.

7. Open your eyes to look at any shoulder.

8. Continue into this position for up to 1 minute.

9. Repeat on the other side.

Two-Knee Spinal Twist

This recovery twist promotes movement and movement in the spine and back. Stretch the spine, back and shoulders. Practicing this pose can help reduce pain and stiffness in the back and hips.

Muscles worked:

1. erector spinae

2. rectus abdominis

3. trapezius

4. large pectoralis

To do this:

1. Lie on your back with your knees pulled to your chest and your arms stretched out to the side.

2. Lower your legs slightly to the left side while keeping your knees as close as possible.

3. You can place a pillow under both knees or between your knees.

4. You can use your left hand to properly press your knees.

5. Keep your neck straight, or turn it to the other side.

6. Focus on breathing deeply in this position.

7. Continue this position for at least 30 seconds.

8. Repeat on the other side.

Child's Pose

This gentle front scroll is a perfect way to relax and release tension in the neck and back. Your spine is stretched and stretched. The Child's Pose also stretches the hips, thighs, and ankles. Practicing this pose can help reduce stress and fatigue.

Muscles worked:

1. gluteus maximus

2. rotator cuff muscles

3. muscles

4. spinal connectors

To do this:

1. Sit on heels and while sitting on the heels your knees should be together.

2. You can use a bolster or dress under your thighs, torso, or forehead for support.

3. Bend forward and move your hands in front of you.

4. Relax your forehead.

5. Keep your arms
    outstretched in front of
    you or bring your arms
    to the side of your
    body with your palms
    facing up.

6. Focus on getting rid of
    tension in your back as
    your upper body falls
    sharply to your knees.

7. continue in this
    position for at most
    five minutes.

**Downward-Facing
Dog (Adho Mukha
Svanasana)**

This yoga helps us to
create a relaxing
mechanism in our

body and also our muscles stretches in different angel. The muscles become reflexive and the chronic pain in the back also in the joints is healed through this yoga.

1. Start by standing straight and fold your palms in the prayer area

2. Insert and raise your arms above your head

3. Exhale and bend slightly and try to touch

the palm of your
hand on the
floor

4. Take a deep
breath and
stretch your left
leg back and
bend your right
knee. Keep your
palms down and
stretch your
fingers

5. Slowly
straighten your
right leg and
make sure your
body is flat on
the floor

6. Bring both
knees down and
take them out.
Relax your
chest, arms and

legs, but lift your
hips to the
ceiling

7. From the
    previous
    position, send
    your elbows to
    the side of your
    body and lift
    your chest up
    and down

8. Switch to a dog
    position facing
    down

9. Insert and bring
    your left foot
    forward

10. Gently lower
    your right foot
    forward, keeping
    your palms in

the same
position

11. Insert and lift
your body and
stretch your
arms above
your head

12. Bring your
hands down
with the palm
facing forward

Sun Salutations (Surya Namaskar)

This is considered to be a body warming up yoga. In this yoga people perform a series of different poses. These poses are performed in a sequence so that a flow could be created. Its other name is Surya Namadkara in

Hinduism. It creates heat in the body and our body gets warm up. It is performed before performing other yoga exercises. It also freshen our minds and we find mind peace while performing this Yoga.

i.   Kneel down, pull inwards forwards

ii.   Stretch your elbows and relax your back

iii.   Stretch your fingers and measure your weight evenly on both palms

iv.   Exhale and lift your knees up and your skin

towards the
ceiling

v.   Stretch your legs gently

vi.   Press down on the heels and palms

vii.   Bring your chest towards our thigh, making sure your shoulders are very open

viii.   Loosen your head and make sure your arms are aligned

ix.   Hold this position for 5-10 breaths

x.   Slowly return to the starting position